I0469461

Altitude Sickness

Altitude Mountain Sickness

Brought To You Courtesy Of:

GetWell Education

GetWell.org

Contributors:

Lara Moore, Editor

Nicolette F. Asselin, M.D., Consultant

References:

National Institute of Health

Altitude Research Institute

American Academy of Family Practice

Center for Disease Control

Legal Disclaimers

This booklet, e-book or app is presented to you for informational purposes only and is not a substitution for any professional advice. The contents herein are based on the views and opinions of the author and all associated contributors.

While every effort has been made by the publisher and all associated contributors to present accurate and up to date information within this document, it is apparent technologies rapidly change. Therefore, the author and all associated contributors reserve the right to update the contents and information provided herein as these changes progress. The author and/or all associated contributors take no responsibility for any errors or omissions if such discrepancies exist within this document.

The authors and all other contributors accept no responsibility for any consequential actions taken, whether monetary, legal, or otherwise, by any and all readers of the materials provided. It is readers sole responsibility to seek professional advice before taking any action on their part.

Readers results will vary based on their skill level and individual perception of the contents herein, and thusly no guarantees, monetarily or otherwise, can be made accurately. Therefore, no guarantees are made.

Manufactured in the United States of America

First Published in 2012

9 7 8 1 4 8 1 0 4 1 9 7 3

Library of Congress Card Number

pending

ISBN: 1481041975
ISBN-13: 978-1481041973
E-Book: pending

DEDICATION

We would like to dedicate this booklet to Family and General Practitioners who have seen their roles as physicians changed tremendously in recent years and struggle with inadequate time to care for their patients.

Index

Foreword

"There is a staggering amount of information available with web resources today. However, I believe that we need to bring things to a basic level to build better understanding and sounder knowledge." N. F. Asselin, M.D.

"Mountains inspire awe in any human person who has a soul. They remind us of our frailty, our unimportance, of the briefness of our span upon this earth. They touch the heavens, and sail serenely at an altitude beyond even the imaginings of a mere mortal." Elizabeth Aston, The Exploits & Adventures of Miss Alethea Darcy, 2005

Acknowledgments

Thank you to everyone on the board for encouraging this publication.
Thank you to Maurice, Sherry Roberts, Judy, Sam, Nick Ramirez, Amy, Sara, and all those involved in the research as well as production of this series

A word from the Editor

The Mission of this series is to offer health prevention resources for the general public. This series has been constructed to have readers achieve a goal by earning points toward a "Health Certificate.

A word from the Consultant

In this series readers will learn to understand the source and prevent illnesses. They will understand the basis as well as be able to recognize symptoms. As a physician, I feel that the information available on the web is a great resource but can become quickly overwhelming and discouraging or produce counterproductive fears to readers.

Mission

GetWell Education mission's:

Is to offer for the general public a basic knowledge on topics that may have a positive effect on their lives.

To prevent unnecessary medical costs and assists people in leading healthier lives.

To empower readers to become an active participant in their care.

To inspire self-respect and knowledge to contribute to reduce health care cost.

To achieve these goals, the team of the Health Series is committed to providing quality education, encompassing personal differences in education and personal background.

The aim is to share information that will encourage self-respect and a sense of dignity rather than anxiety or avoidance of health issues.

Chapter 1 Introduction

It may be harmful to your health not to know about this topic! On the other hand, you may already know what we are about to share with you.

Before you read this book

1. Take the Quiz on the back of this booklet. If you score a 100% move to level 2 series. If you score less than that, read the booklet and take the quiz again at the end.

2. It is important that you choose a time when you can relax so you can retain the important facts you are about to read. Now a day, we are so bombarded with information that it is, at time, difficult to remember simple things. Less is better.

3. This booklet is the building block on which you will construct important life changing behaviors as well as learn to recognize life-changing information.

Notes:

Score before reading: ______

Score after reading: ______

Chapter 2 Definition

What is Altitude Sickness?

The stresses of the high-altitude environment include cold, low humidity, increased ultraviolet radiation, and decreased air pressure, all of which can cause problems for travelers. The largest concern, however, is hypoxia. At 10,000 ft (3,000 m), for example, the inspired PO2 is only 69% of sea-level value. The degree of hypoxic stress depends on altitude, rate of ascent, and duration of exposure. Sleeping at high altitude produces the most hypoxia; day trips to high altitude with return to low altitude are much less stressful on the body. Typical high-altitude destinations include Cuzco (11,000 ft; 3,300 m), La Paz (12,000 ft; 3,640 m), Lhasa (12,100 ft; 3,650 m), Everest Base Camp (17,700 ft; 5,400 m), and Kilimanjaro (19,341ft; 5,895 m).

The human body adjusts very well to moderate hypoxia, but requires time to do so (Box 2-02). The process of acute acclimatization to high altitude takes 3–5 days; therefore, acclimatizing for a few days at 8,000–9,000 ft before proceeding to a higher altitude is ideal. Acclimatization prevents altitude illness, improves sleep, and increases comfort and well-being, although exercise performance will always be reduced compared with low altitude. Increase in ventilation is the most important factor in acute acclimatization; therefore, respiratory depressants must be avoided. Increased red-cell production does not play a role in acute acclimatization.

Reference: Peter H. Hackett, David R. Shlim

How is it determined?

Altitude sickness is determined by observation and paying close attention to your symptoms.

(see chapter 3)

What are the risks?

RISK FOR TRAVELERS

Inadequate acclimatization may lead to altitude illness in any traveler going to 8,000 ft (2,500 m) or higher. Susceptibility and resistance to altitude illness are genetic traits, and no screening tests are available to predict risk. Risk is not affected by training or physical fitness. Children are equally susceptible as adults; people aged >50 years have slightly lower risk. How a traveler has responded to high altitude previously is the most reliable guide for future trips, but is not infallible. However, given certain baseline susceptibility, risk is largely influenced by rate of ascent and exertion (see Table 2-06). Determining an itinerary that will avoid any occurrence of altitude illness is difficult because of variations in individual susceptibility, as well as in starting points and terrain. (1)

Summary:

Altitude sickness is a serious condition. If ignored certain aspect can be fatal.

Reference

1) Peter H. Hackett, David R. Shlim, Center for Disease Control and Prevention

Chapter 3 Symptoms

How do I know I have Altitude Sickness (AS)?

Altitude illness is divided into 3 syndromes:

1. AMS

Altitude Mountain Sickness

AMS is the most common form of altitude illness, affecting, for example, 25% of all visitors sleeping above 8,000 ft (2,500 m) in Colorado.

Symptoms: Symptoms are those of an alcohol hangover: headache is the cardinal symptom, sometimes accompanied by fatigue, loss of appetite, nausea, and occasionally vomiting.

Headache onset is usually 2–12 hours after arrival at a higher altitude and often during or after the first night.

* Preverbal children may develop loss of appetite, irritability, and pallor.

Solution: AMS generally resolves with 24–72 hours of acclimatization.

2. HACE

High Altitude Cerebral Edema

HACE is a severe progression of AMS and is rare; it is most often associated with HAPE.

Symptoms: In addition to AMS symptoms, lethargy becomes profound, with drowsiness, confusion, and ataxia on tandem gait test.

Solution: A person with HACE requires immediate descent; death from HACE can ensue within 24 hours of developing ataxia, if the person fails to descend.

Notes:

3. HAPE

High Altitude Pulmonary Edema

HAPE can occur by itself or in conjunction with AMS and HACE; incidence is 1 per 10,000 skiers in Colorado and up to 1 per 100 climbers at more than 14,000 ft (4,270 m).

Symptoms: Initial symptoms are increased breathlessness with exertion, and eventually increased breathlessness at rest, associated with weakness and cough.

Solution: Oxygen or descent is life-saving. HAPE can be more rapidly fatal than HACE.

Notes:

Quick Reference

Conditions	Symptoms
AMS	Severe headache that is not relieved by medication Nausea and vomiting, increasing weakness and fatigue Shortness of breath
HACE	Headache Weakness Disorientation Loss of co-ordination Decreasing levels of consciousness Loss of memory Hallucinations & Psychotic behavior Decreased co-ordination (ataxia). Coma
HAPE	Shortness of breath at rest Tightness in the chest, and a persistent cough bringing up white, watery, or frothy fluid Marked fatigue and weakness A feeling of impending suffocation at night Confusion, and irrational behavior

Chapter 4 Cause

What is the Cause of Primary AS?

Cause

All forms of altitude sickness are caused by low levels of oxygen at very high altitudes.

Going too high too quickly

These lower levels result in hypoxia, a shortage of oxygen in the body's tissues. The effects of hypoxia may be mild or even unnoticeable. Altitude sickness is most likely to occur with a rapid increase in elevation, as well as by the cold experienced at high altitudes.

People can adjust to the effects of hypoxia at high altitudes, but only up to a point. At elevations up to 3,000 meters (10,000 feet), most people have no problems after a few days. But no one can survive permanently above 5,100 meters (17,000 feet). At the elevations reached by mountain climbers, bottled oxygen often becomes necessary.

Acclimatization

The main cause of altitude sickness is going too high too quickly. Given enough time, your body will adapt to the decrease in oxygen at a specific altitude. This process is known as acclimatization and generally takes one to three days at any given altitude, e.g. if you climb to 3,000 meters and spend several days at that altitude, your body will acclimatize to 3,000 meters. If you then climb to 5,000 meters your body has to acclimatize once again.

Several changes take place in the body that enables it to cope with decreased oxygen:

- The depth of respiration increases.
- The body produces more red blood cells to carry oxygen.
- Pressure in pulmonary capillaries is increased, "forcing" blood into parts of the lung that are not normally used when breathing at sea level.
- The body produces more of a particular enzyme that causes the release of oxygen from hemoglobin to the body tissues.
-

Risk Factors

Travelers with medical conditions, such as heart failure, myocardial ischemia (angina), sickle cell disease, or any form of **pulmonary insufficiency**, should be advised to consult a physician familiar with high-altitude medical issues before undertaking high-altitude travel.

The risk for new ischemic heart disease in previously healthy travelers does not appear to be increased at high altitudes. People with diabetes can travel safely to high altitudes, but they must be accustomed to exercise and carefully monitor their blood glucose. Diabetic ketoacidosis may be triggered by altitude illness and may be more difficult to treat in those on acetazolamide.

Not all glucose meters read accurately at high altitudes.

Most people do not have visual problems at high altitudes. However, at very high altitudes some people who have had radial keratotomy may develop acute farsightedness and be unable to climb by themselves. LASIK and other newer procedures may produce only minor visual disturbances at high altitudes.

There are no studies or case reports of harm to a fetus if the mother travels briefly to high altitudes during pregnancy. However, it may be prudent to recommend that pregnant women do not stay at sleeping altitudes higher than 12,000 ft (3,658 m), if possible. The dangers of having a pregnancy complication in remote, mountainous terrain should also be discussed.

Chapter 5 Prevention

How can I Prevent Severe Altitude Illness or death?

Preventative steps

The main point about altitude illness is not to eliminate the possibility, but to prevent death or evacuation due to altitude sickness. Since the onset of symptoms and the clinical course are sufficiently slow and predictable, there is no reason for someone to die from altitude illness, unless trapped by weather or geography in a situation in which descent is impossible.

Three rules can prevent death or serious consequences from altitude illness:

- Know the early symptoms of altitude illness, and be willing to acknowledge when they are present.
- Never ascend to sleep at a higher altitude when experiencing symptoms of altitude illness, no matter how minor they seem.
- Descend if the symptoms become worse while resting at the same altitude.

Note: For trekking groups and expeditions going into remote high-altitude areas, where descent to a lower altitude could be problematic, a pressurization bag (such as the Gamow bag) can be beneficial.

Incidence

Most people can ascend to 1500 to 2000 m (5000 to 6500 ft) in one day without problems, but about 20% of those who ascend to 2500 m (8000 ft) and 40% of those who ascend to 3000 m (10,000 ft) develop some form of AS. Rate of ascent, maximum altitude reached, and sleeping altitude influence the likelihood of developing the disorder.

Risk factors

Effects of high altitude vary greatly among individuals. Going too high too fast

But generally, risk is increased by:

- Exertion
- Risk is greater in people who have had previous AS and in those who live at low altitude (< 900 m [< 3000 ft]).
- Young children and young adults are probably more susceptible.

- Disorders such as diabetes, coronary artery disease, and mild COPD are not risk factors for AS, but hypoxia may adversely affect these disorders.
- Physical fitness is not protective.

How well do older persons tolerate moderate altitude?

Effects of high altitude do not vary with age and has been tested to be lower in older adults.

HACE and HAPE are life threatening

every seconds counts.

Returning to lower level and seeking medical help is crucial.

Chapter 6 Preventative Approach

Are there any preventative treatments?

Preventative Medications

Acetazolamide (Diamox)

This is the most tried and tested drug for altitude sickness prevention and treatment.

Unlike dexamethasone this drug does not mask the symptoms but actually treats the problem. It seems to works by increasing the amount of alkali (bicarbonate) excreted in the urine, making the blood more acidic. Acidifying the blood drives the ventilation (breathing), which is the cornerstone of acclimatization.

For prevention, typically physicians will prescribe 125 to 250mg twice daily. Starting one or two days before and continuing for three days once the highest altitude is reached, is effective. Blood concentrations of the medicine will be highest between one to four hours after taking the tablets.

A trial course is recommended

Gradual ascent is always desirable to try to avoid acute mountain sickness. However, if rapid ascent is undertaken and that acetazolamide is used, it should be noted if severe forms of high altitude sickness occur such as pulmonary or cerebral edema (HACE and HAPE), that the need for a prompt descent still is still most advisable.

Side effects of acetazolamide include: an uncomfortable tingling of the fingers, toes and face carbonated drinks tasting flat; excessive urination; and rarely, blurring of vision. In case of mountain climbing, gradual ascent is possible and prophylaxis tends to be discouraged.

Note: A trial course is recommended before going to a remote location where a severe allergic reaction could prove difficult to treat if it occurred.

Dexamethasone

Dexamethasone (a steroid) is a drug that decreases swelling of the brain and other area. It reverses the effects of AMS but does not treat the problem. The dose is typically 4 mg twice a day for a few days starting with the ascent. This alleviate most of the symptoms of altitude illness.

WARNING: Dexamethasone is a powerful drug and should be used with caution and only on the advice of a physician. It should only be used to aid acclimatization under supervision of qualified persons with the necessary experience of its use.

How do I know that these medications will not do me more harm than good?

It is important to have a dialogue with your physician. Certain medicines do not work for every one.

Again, a trial course is recommended before going to a remote location where a severe allergic reaction could prove difficult to treat if it occurred.

Chapter 7 for Professionals

Pathophysiology

Acute hypoxia (e.g., as occurs during rapid ascent to high altitude in an unpressurized aircraft) alters CNS function within minutes. However, AS results from the body's neurohumoral and hemodynamic responses to hypoxia and develops over hours to days.

The CNS and lungs are primarily affected. In both, elevated capillary pressure, capillary leakage, and consequent edema formation probably occurs.

In the lungs, hypoxia-induced elevation of pulmonary artery pressure causes interstitial and alveolar pulmonary edema, resulting in impaired oxygenation.

Small-vessel hypoxic vasoconstriction is patchy, causing over perfusion with elevated pressure, capillary wall damage, and capillary leakage in less constricted areas. Various additional mechanisms have been proposed; they include sympathetic over activity, endothelial dysfunction, decreased alveolar nitric oxide (perhaps due to decreased nitric oxide synthase), and a defect in the amiloride-sensitive Na channel. Some of these factors may have a genetic component.

Pathophysiology in the CNS is less clear but may involve a combination of hypoxia-induced cerebral vasodilatation, alteration of the blood-brain barrier, and Na and water retention causing cerebral edema. One hypothesis is that patients with a low ratio of CSF to brain volume are less able to tolerate swelling (i.e., by displacement of CSF) and thus are more likely to develop AS. The roles of atrial natriuretic peptide, aldosterone, renin, and angiotensin are unclear.

Diagnosis

Clinical evaluation

Diagnosis of most forms of AS is clinical; laboratory tests are nonspecific and usually unnecessary. HACE can usually be differentiated from other causes of coma (e.g., infection, ketoacidosis) by the history and by absence of fever and nuchal rigidity. If done, blood and CSF studies are normal. In HAPE, hypoxemia is often severe, with pulse oximetry showing 40 to 70%

saturation. If obtained, chest x-ray shows a normal-sized heart and patchy lung edema (often middle or lower lobes), unlike what is seen in heart failure.

Prevention

Studies have shown that taking this preventative medicine at a dose of 250mg every eight to twelve hours (2-3 times/day) before and during rapid ascent to altitude results in fewer and/or less severe symptoms (such as headache, nausea, shortness of breath, dizziness, drowsiness, and fatigue) of acute mountain sickness (AMS). Pulmonary function is greater both in people who have no symptoms or with mild AMS. The climbers who took the medicine also had less difficulty sleeping.

In case of mountain climbing, gradual ascent is possible and prophylaxis tends to be discouraged. However, if climbers do develop headache and nausea or the other symptoms of AMS, then treatment with acetazolamide is fine. The typical treatment dosage is 250 mg twice a day for about three days.

Patients who have had a previous episode of HAPE should consider prophylaxis with sustained-release nifedipine 20 to 30 mg po bid. Inhaled β-agonists may also be effective.

Gradual ascent is always desirable to try to avoid acute mountain sickness. However, if rapid ascent is undertaken and acetazolamide is used, it should be noted if severe forms of high altitude sickness occur, i.e. pulmonary or cerebral edema, that the need for a prompt descent still is still advisable.

Treatment

For mild or moderate AMS, halting ascent and treatment with fluids, analgesics, and sometimes acetazolamide

For severe symptoms, immediate descent and treatment with O2, drugs, and pressurization

AMS

Patients should halt ascent and reduce exertion until symptoms resolve. Other treatment includes fluids and analgesics for headache. For severe symptoms, descent of 500 to 1000 m (1650 to 3200 ft) is usually rapidly effective. Acetazolamide 250 mg po bid may relieve symptoms and improve sleep.

HAPE & HACE

Patients should descend to low altitude immediately. If descent is delayed, patients should rest and be given O2. If descent is impossible, O2, drugs, and pressurization in a portable hyperbaric bag help buy time but are not substitutes for descent.

HAPE: For HAPE, nifedipine 10 mg sublingually followed by a 30-mg slow-release tablet lowers pulmonary artery pressure and is beneficial. Diuretics (e.g., furosemide) are contraindicated. The heart is normal in HAPE, and digitalis is of no value. When promptly treated by descent, patients usually recover from HAPE within 24 to 48 h. People who have had one episode of HAPE are likely to have another and should be so warned.

HACE: For HACE (and severe AMS), dexamethasone 4 to 8 mg initially, followed by 4 mg q 6 h, may help. It may be given po, sc, IM, or IV. Acetazolamide 250 mg po bid may be added.

Prevention

The most important measure is a slow ascent. Drinking extra water is important because breathing large volumes of dry air at altitude greatly increases water loss, and dehydration with some degree of hypovolemia aggravates symptoms. Alcohol seems to worsen AMS and reduces nocturnal ventilation, thus accentuating sleep disturbance. Although physical fitness enables greater exertion at altitude, it does not protect against any form of AS.

Older Adults

A study done in Vail, Colorado, at an elevation of 2,500 m (8,200 ft) that the incidence of acute mountain sickness was 16%, which is slightly lower than that reported for younger persons. The occurrence of symptoms of acute mountain sickness did not parallel arterial oxygen saturation or spirometric or blood pressure measurements. Chronic diseases were present in percentages typical for ambulatory elderly persons: 19 (20%) had coronary artery disease, 33 (34%) had hypertension, and 9 (9%) had lung disease. Despite this, no adverse signs or symptoms occurred in our subjects during their stay at this altitude. Our findings suggest that persons with preexisting, generally asymptomatic, cardiovascular or pulmonary disease can safely visit moderate altitudes.

Three rules can prevent death or serious consequences from altitude illness (page 20)

Ascent

Graded ascent is essential for activity at > 2500 m (> 8000 ft). Sleeping on the first night should be at < 2500 to 3000 m (8,000 to 10,000 ft), and climbers should sleep at that altitude for 2 to 3 nights if subsequent higher sleeping altitudes are planned. Each day thereafter, sleeping altitude can be increased by about 300 m (1000 ft), although higher day hikes are acceptable with return to the lower level for sleep. Climbers vary in ability to ascend without developing symptoms; a climbing party should be paced for its slowest member.

Acclimatization reverses quickly

Acclimatization reverses quickly. After descent to low levels for more than a few days, acclimatized climbers should once more follow a graded ascent.

Drugs

Acetazolamide 125 to 250 mg po q 12 h reduces the incidence of AMS. Sustained-release capsules (500 mg once/day) are also available. Acetazolamide can be started on the day of the ascent; it acts by inhibiting carbonic anhydrase and thus increasing ventilation. Acetazolamide 125 mg by mouth at bedtime reduces the amount of periodic breathing (almost universal during sleep at high altitude), thus limiting sharp falls in blood O2.

Counter indication:

Acetazolamide should not be given to patients ***allergic to sulfa drugs***. Analogs of acetazolamide offer no advantage.

O2:

Low-flow O2 during sleep at altitude is effective but inconvenient and may pose logistic difficulties.

Side effects and problems:

Acetazolamide may cause numbness and fingers paresthesia; these symptoms are benign but can be annoying. Carbonated drinks taste flat to people taking acetazolamide. Dexamethasone 2 mg po q 6 h is an alternative to acetazolamide. However, there is a risk of masking symptoms.

With treatment for longer than 48 hours, we recommend Potassium rich dietary supplement such as bananas or Gatorade.

Recommended medication doses for prevention of altitude illness

MEDICATION	INDICATION	ROUTE	DOSE
Acetazolamide	**AMS,HACE** prevention	Oral	125 mg Q2D Pediatrics: 2.5 mg/kg every 12 h
Dexamethasone (with caution)	**AMS, HACE** prevention	Oral	2 mg every 6 h or 4 mg every 12 h Pediatrics: should not be used for prophylaxis

Recommended medication doses to for treatment of altitude illness

Consult Emergency Manual

Chapter 8 Facts

About 1 in 5 US adults have Altitude sickness over 2500 m (8000ft) and 2 out of 5 at 3000 m (10,000 ft)

Rate of ascent, maximum altitude reached, and sleeping altitude influence the likelihood of developing the disorder.

Your role is important

Do I have altitude sickness?

Altitude sickness, also called Altitude Mountain Sickness (AMS) is a combination of symptoms that are present when your body does not adapt to its current altitude. The most frequent symptoms of AMS are headache, queasiness, tiredness and trouble sleeping.

Am I at risk of developing AMS?

Anyone who goes to altitude can get AMS, despite age, gender, physical fitness, or previous altitude experience. If you know from previous experience that you are susceptible to AMS, there are steps you can take to prevent it.

What can I do to prevent AMS?

You can greatly reduce the symptoms of AMS by asking your doctor for a prescription drug called acetazolamide (Diamox). If you are not sure if you are susceptible, but want to optimize your experience at altitude, we recommend you:

- Avoid going directly to a sleeping altitude of over 9,000 ft in one day
- Consider adding a day at a modest altitude such as Denver (5,000 to 6,000 feet)

Once at higher altitudes we recommend you:

- Drink more fluids and less alcohol
- Eat less salty foods
- Take it easy for the first day or two

When to seek medical help?

If your symptoms get worse or do not go away after a day or two at altitude, you need to seek medical help. All medical centers in altitude communities are used to dealing with these symptoms.

My heart seems to beat faster, is this normal?

On arrival at altitude many people notice that they are more breathless and their heart beats faster, especially when they exert themselves. These are your body's normal, early responses to altitude adaptation.

I am in very good physical shape – doesn't that mean that I'm less likely to feel the effects of the altitude?

Being physically fit does not prevent you from experiencing AMS symptoms. There does not seem to be a link between fitness level and susceptibility to altitude illness.

I have a mild headache – is it safe to take Tylenol?

You can take one or two tablets of Tylenol, aspirin, or ibuprofen. You can buy those at a drug store.

Age - should I worry more about feeling poorly because I am older?

Actually, older people seem to be less susceptible to AMS.

I know I don't feel well when I get to higher elevations – is there a prescription I can take?

You can ask your doctor for acetazolamide (Diamox), a prescription drug that alleviates AMS symptoms. Known side effects include: increased urinary output, a tingling sensation in fingers and toes. It also makes carbonated beverages taste flat. If you're allergic to sulfa drugs you should not take Diamox.

Are there any over the counter drugs / herbal remedies that counteract the effects of altitude?

There are some studies that suggest Gingko Biloba may decrease AMS symptoms in some individuals.

What warning signals should I be aware of?

Warning signals of AMS are: headache, queasy stomach, tiredness and trouble sleeping. Symptoms lasting more than a couple of days, difficulty breathing at rest, loss of coordination, or extreme listlessness are signs you need to seek immediate medical attention.

I am pregnant – is it safe for me to go to higher elevations?

Travel to moderate altitude (8,000-12,000 feet) is not a problem in pregnancy. However the terrain for skiers and hikers may be a problem for some women later in pregnancy.

What about children at altitude?

Children also get symptoms of AMS. In the very young pre-verbal children this may manifest in fussiness, decreased appetite and trouble sleeping.

I have high blood pressure – is it safe for me to go to higher elevations?

Blood pressure levels do increase the first few days at moderate altitudes. If you know you have high blood pressure and take medication for this, it may be advisable to check it once or twice after arrival at altitude to see if your medication requires adjustment. Remember if you increase your meds at altitude, you may need to decrease them again when you return home.

I have heart disease / lung disease - is it safe for me to go to high altitude?

Some people with chronic lung conditions may require oxygen when traveling to altitude. It is best to check with your own doctor for advice. Some people with heart problems like angina may get more heart pains in the first day or two before they adapt. Others who have had stents or bypass surgery may do just fine. Give our altitude clinic a call for a consultation on your condition.

I just got to the mountains last night and am feeling queasy – what should I do?

Queasiness is a common symptom of AMS. It will usually pass in 24-36 hours. Avoiding alcohol and eating foods that are easy to digest may be helpful.

I've planned a party on my first night at altitude - should I?

It is best to wait until you have adapted to altitude before you party. The combination of alcohol, the dry air and altitude may make you feel more tired and dehydrated the next day.

I feel more tired that I expected - should I take it easy - for how long?

Feeling tired is a common symptom of altitude adaptation. Your symptoms should go away in 24-36 hours.

I have trouble sleeping and keep waking up at night.

This is one of the more common symptoms of altitude exposure. Your sleep will improve with each night you stay. If it continues you can use low doses of acetazolamide (Diamox) to help you sleep.

Ref. Altitude Sickness Research Center,
University of Colorado

Chapter 9 Quiz

Test Your AS IQ with this quiz:

Gazing down on the spectacular view from a mountaintop can take your breath away. That breathlessness is oftentimes more than just an awestruck reaction to the sights. It can be a symptom of altitude sickness, an illness that can strike hikers, mountain climbers, skiers, and anyone who hits the 8,000-foot mark on a mountain. Learn more about this condition by taking this true-false quiz.

1. Altitude sickness is also called mountain sickness.
A. True
B. False

2. If you live close to sea level, you are more likely to feel the effects of high altitude when visiting high places.
A. True
B. False

3. Altitude sickness occurs because a person on a mountain is so much closer to the sun than at sea level.

A. True
B. False

4. In severe cases of altitude sickness, fluid collects in the lungs and the brain swells.
A. True
B. False

5. If you notice mild symptoms of altitude sickness, it's fine to keep on climbing.
A. True
B. False

6. People with severe emphysema or chronic obstructive pulmonary disease shouldn't travel to high elevations.
A. True
B. False

Answers

1. Altitude sickness is also called mountain sickness.
You answered A. True.
The correct answer is A. True.

Other names for this illness include altitude anoxia; more serious forms are called high altitude pulmonary edema and high altitude cerebral edema.

2. If you live close to sea level, you are more likely to feel the effects of high altitude when visiting high places.
You answered A. True.
The correct answer is A. True.

Children also are more likely to feel the effects of high altitude. One way to prevent altitude sickness is to ascend heights gradually. Take several days to move up to 8,000 feet. Beyond that height, don't climb any faster than about 1,000 feet a day. Experts also recommend sleeping at a lower altitude than you spend the day at. If you're climbing, for instance, don't make camp at the highest point you've reached for the day, but backtrack down the trail at least several hundred feet.

3. Altitude sickness occurs because a person on a mountain is so much closer to the sun than at sea level.
You answered B. False.

The correct answer is B. False.

Altitude sickness occurs because the higher up you go; the less oxygen is in the air for you to breathe. It occurs most commonly at elevations above 8,000 feet. If you live in the mountains, your body adapts. At 14,000 feet and above, however, nearly everyone experiences at least mild symptoms of altitude sickness.

4. In severe cases of altitude sickness, fluid collects in the lungs and the brain swells.

You answered A. True.

The correct answer is A. True.

These are life-threatening conditions and require immediate medical care. Milder symptoms include shortness of breath, trouble sleeping, headache, insomnia, nausea, rapid pulse, fatigue, and dizziness. More serious symptoms include coughing, tightness in the chest, difficulty walking in a straight line, and mental confusion.

5. If you notice mild symptoms of altitude sickness, it's fine to keep on climbing.

You answered B. False.

The correct answer is B. False.

If you notice even mild symptoms, don't go any higher. If you have symptoms of altitude sickness, it's important that you return to a lower elevation. For example, if you are at an altitude of 8,000 to 9,000 feet, you may need to travel down to an elevation of 6,000 feet or lower for your symptoms to go away. A health care provider may prescribe medications to prevent or treat the symptoms of severe high altitude sickness. If your symptoms go away at a lower altitude, you may try to return to a higher elevation after your body adjusts. This may take one to three days.

6. People with severe emphysema or chronic obstructive pulmonary disease shouldn't travel to high elevations.

You answered A. True.

The correct answer is A. True.

You also should avoid high elevations if you have severe heart disease or sickle cell anemia. If you have mild heart or lung disease, and you are managing it well, you might be fine at high elevations. Check with your health care provider to see if it's safe.

Evaluation:

If your score is: 100% you may move to level 2 booklet.

If your score is lower, read this booklet and take the quiz again.

www.ingramcontent.com/pod-product-compliance
Lightning Source LLC
Chambersburg PA
CBHW071728170526
45165CB00005B/2201
9781481041973